Holsman
Physical Therapy
& Rehabilitation P.C.

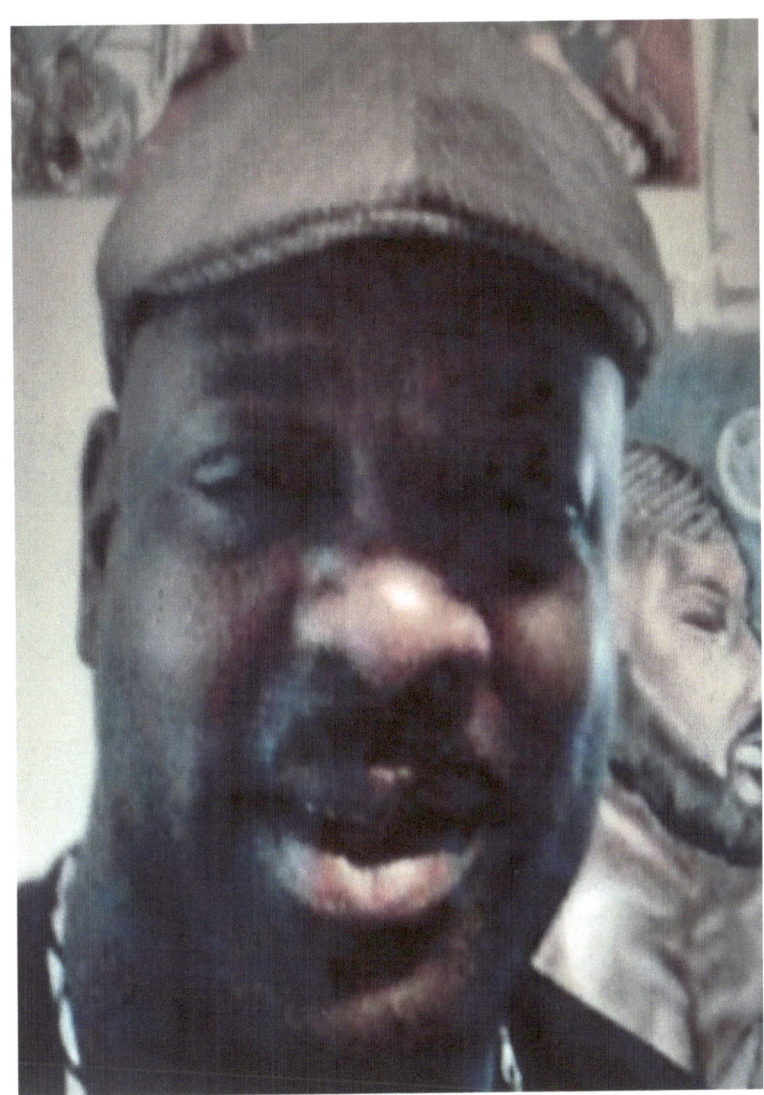

I'm Walking Again

Through Physical Therapy

I was diagnosed with a Gout and Arthritis symptoms in the year 2000. I was working at Passaic County College in Paterson NJ, as an in-house staff security officer. My job was to transport money from Passaic County College to a bank escorted by Paterson Police Department. After my duty and shifted was over I started to feel some stiffness in both of my legs, it got tighter and tighter. It became totally unbearable to walk or sit. As the doctor checked my blood, vital signs etc, he said it's from all that rich man's eating, which was spicy food. I was given some medicine at that time that I didn't kept up with and things only got worse, every year or more I started to get gout, arthritis in my hands and arms, swollen as fast in seconds. I felt pain as no one has before, from the slightest touch. I was then given something for the pain.

There is one thing I want you to know about pain medication". Whatever pain medication they give you for pain, read up on it. But not to worry you will be relieved of the pain temporarily, until the next time you don't watch you're eating habits. By you taking pain killers to relieve your pain, you are missing out on something more important, that only the x-ray can see, oh you can feel it. X-ray shows the wear and tear of bone against bone, **bone against bone causing (Uric Acid) to develop.**

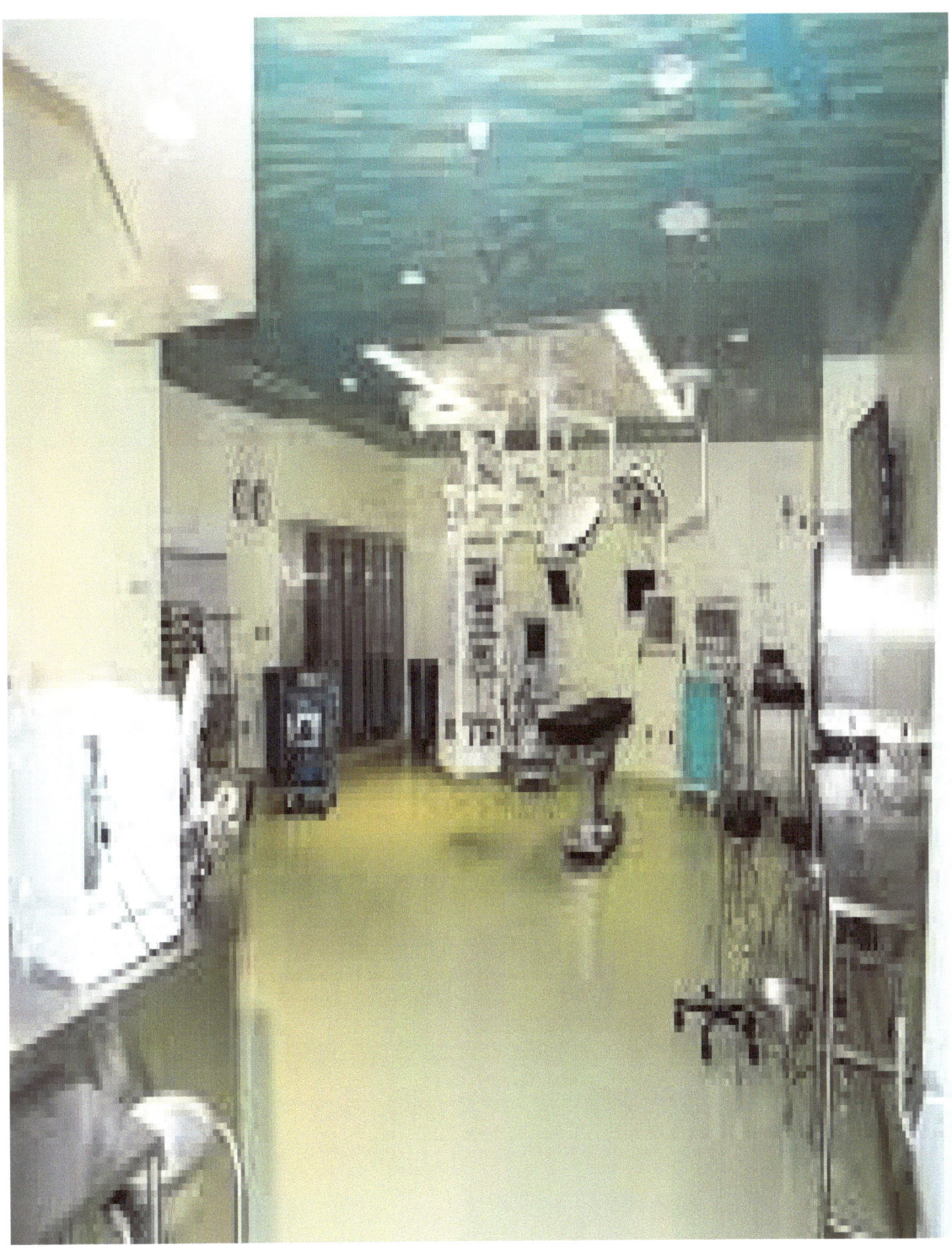

This is one of the operating room at Mountainside Hospital. On July3rd, 2016

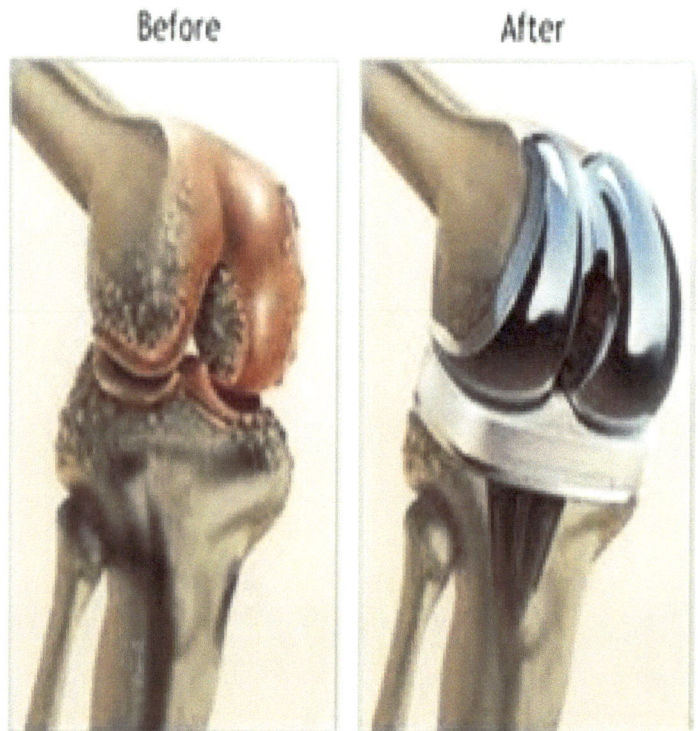

Before   After

My Orthopedic surgeon had given me
Options; he said he could drain the inflammation out of your
knee. But it would just keep coming back, so I had decided to
get the knee transplant. I truly didn't want to feel that kind of
pain again year after year or even month after month. My
knees were weak and I needed his help.

Still I had to get the knees drained out before surgery. He used a large clear tube syringe, and stuck it in my knee to abstract it out.

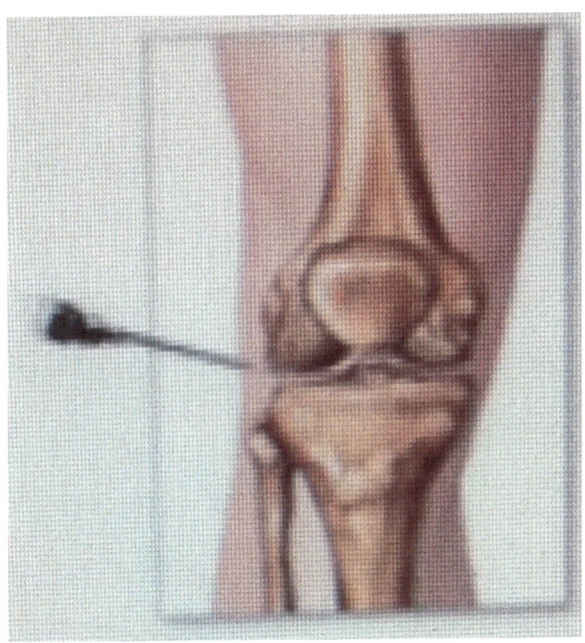

My situation was very serious; as he pull out the uric acid I seen the gold like yellow, liquid crystal being drained out. After that I was given pain medication.

You can ask the doctor's advice on pain medication, he would be glad to help you. Tylenol Arthritis, really don't work for most people, but the Ibuprofen does for some. For the most part you want to feel better. All medicine you use, you must eat something first before taking it.

- 1st hour: When I woke up I didn't feel any pain, just a little stiffness, temporarily.
- I was hooked up to different devices, medication going directly into the leg area. The other was taking out wasteful fluid that caused the swelling. There were tubes for everything, even for the restroom.
- It was recommended Physical Therapy the second and third day, where I walked to the front desk.
- Pain medication should be taken before each session of physical therapy and before you go to sleep each night so that you can sleep peaceful.
- 3rd day there is no pain in your leg. You will be going to a physical therapy recreational center for patients, working on yourself and keeping a steady diet.
- Ice will be your best friend to take down most of the swelling ,use an ace bandage and wrap it up daily
- I've been in physical therapy for a couple of months, but not fully walking yet on my own.
- My way getting around was mainly the wheel chair. The crutches and walkers didn't come until later.

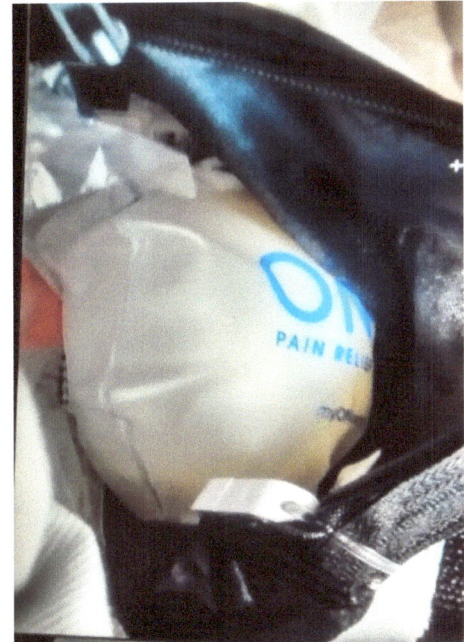

1st

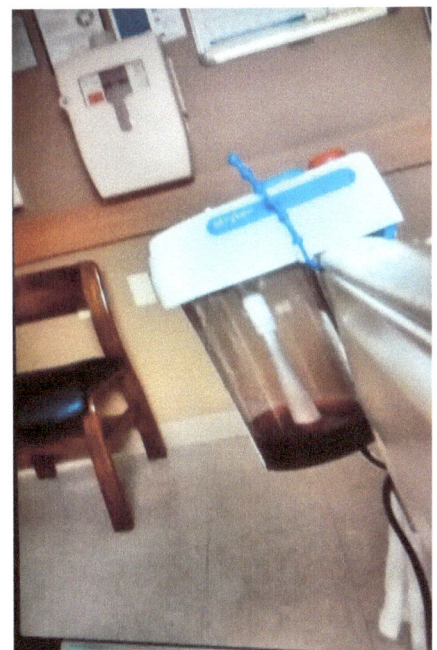

2nd

1st You will be hooked up with some of these things here is a medicine bag for the pain that is going directly into your leg by tube that will be attached to your surgery , the nurse can turn it up or down for more pain relief medicine to go into your leg. 2nd Is fluid that has to come out of your leg so that you are able to bend and heal right. 3rd This is a machine that is to prevent any form of blood clots from performing within this leg, they have warm censors on it

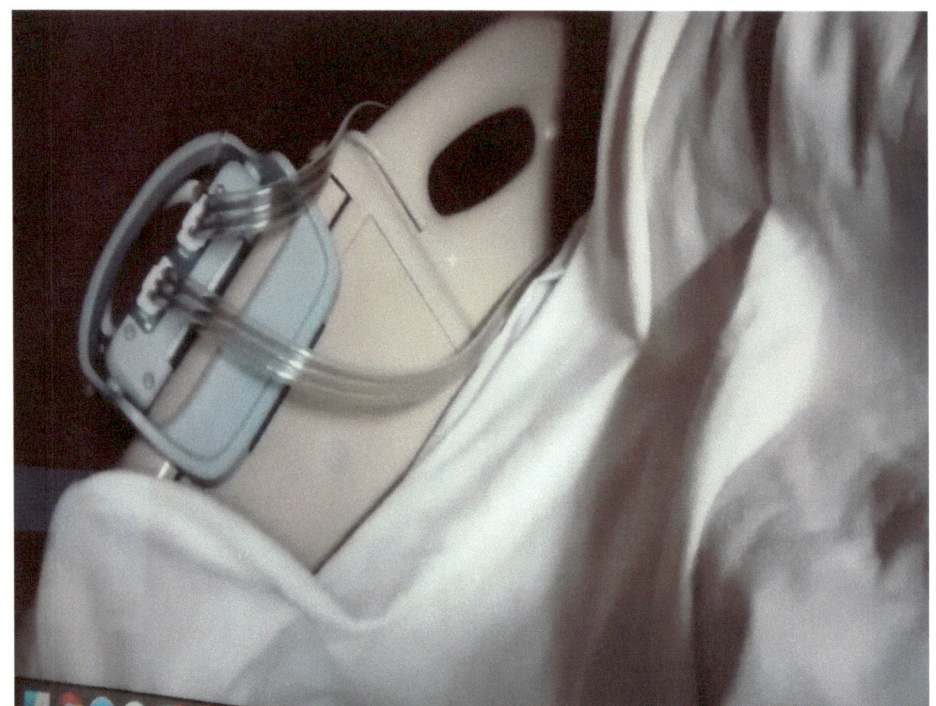

3rd

You are scrapped into this machine to prevent blood clots

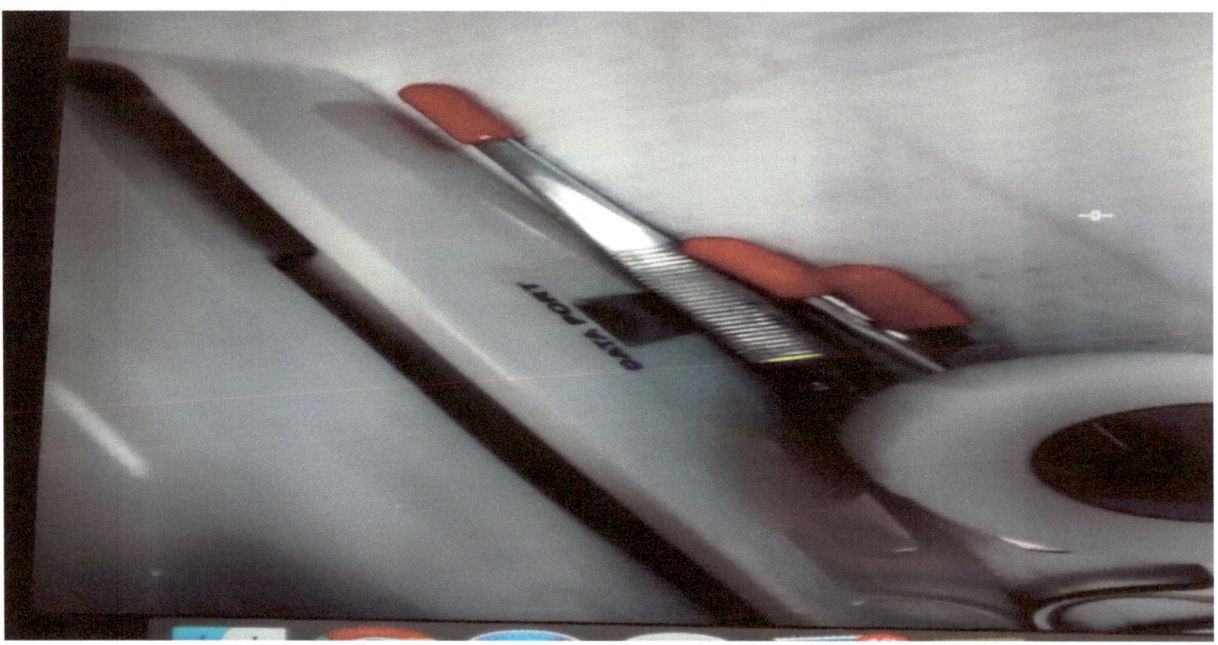

The third day the bandages comes off.

The hospital showed me a list of food that I should pay attention to, because it can prevent gout from spreading through your body. I thought that it was very useful.

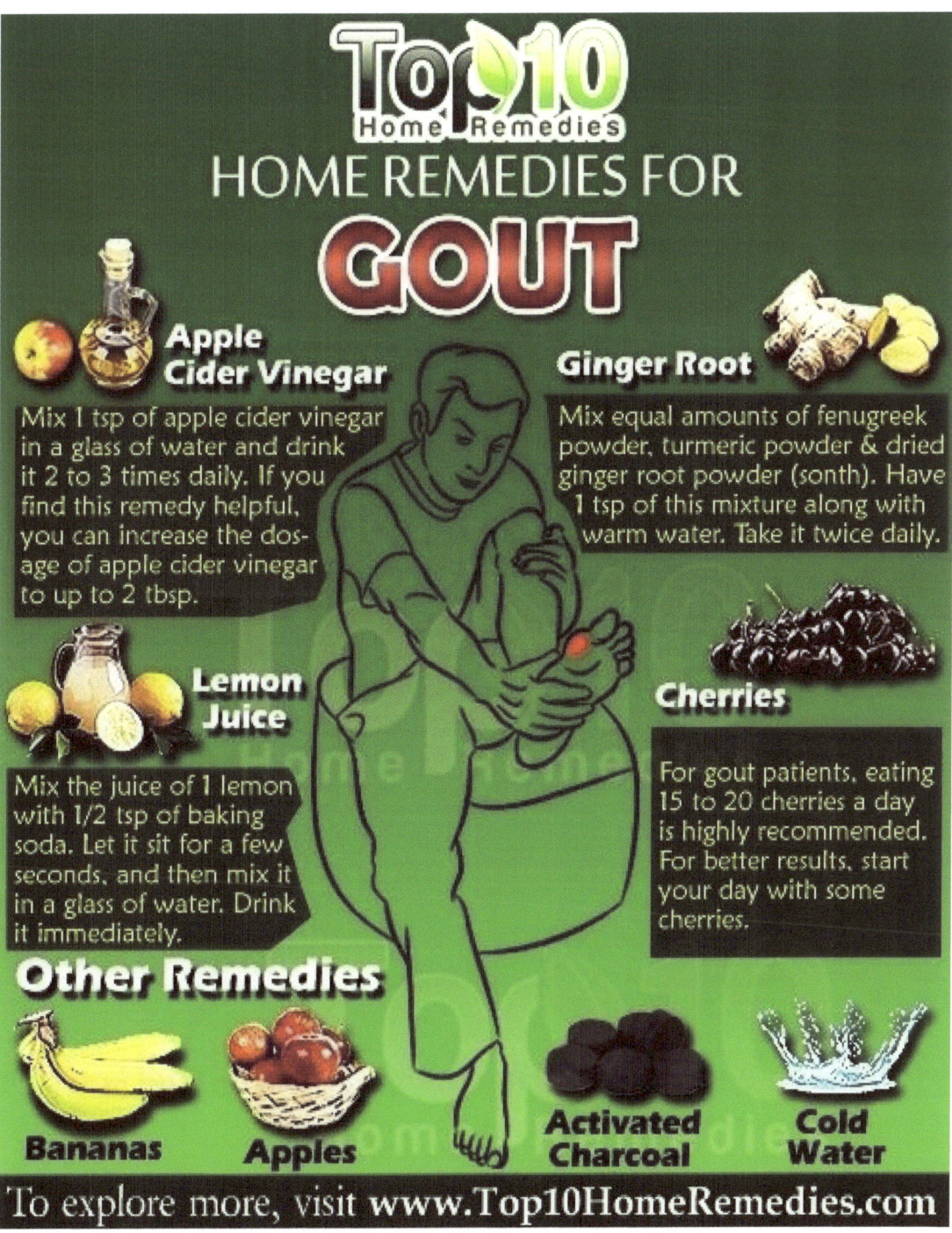

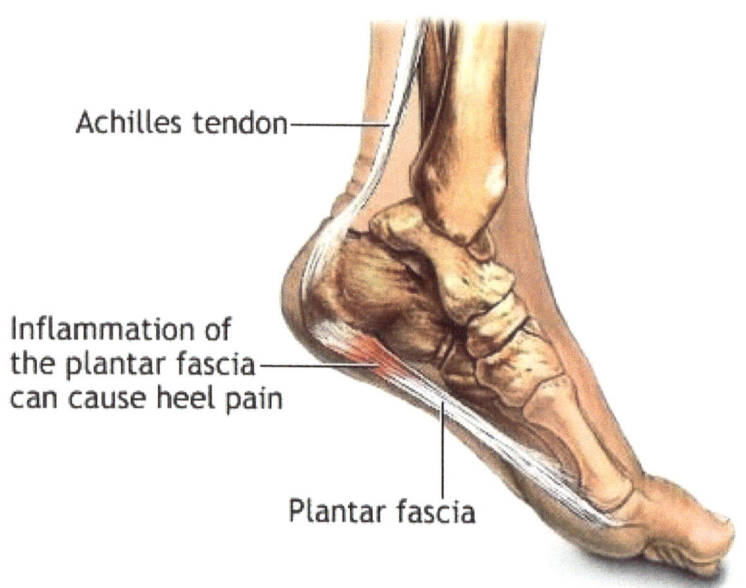

Achilles tendon

Inflammation of
the plantar fascia
can cause heel pain

Plantar fascia

Even though I had the operation on my knee, I still had gout in my feet. This is where it difficult for me to walk I had to lose weight and plus eat right, and plenty of physical therapy. I started to make big changes in my life that was beneficial to me.

I then went to a podiatrist in Englewood NJ, who had helped me get back on my feet also. But the real job was through physical therapy, you would have to walk on these feet and also stand and exercise.

Inserts of your shoes or sneakers where made, molded for your comfort.

My next step was to go to Holsman's Physical Therapy on my release date: July 28, 2016

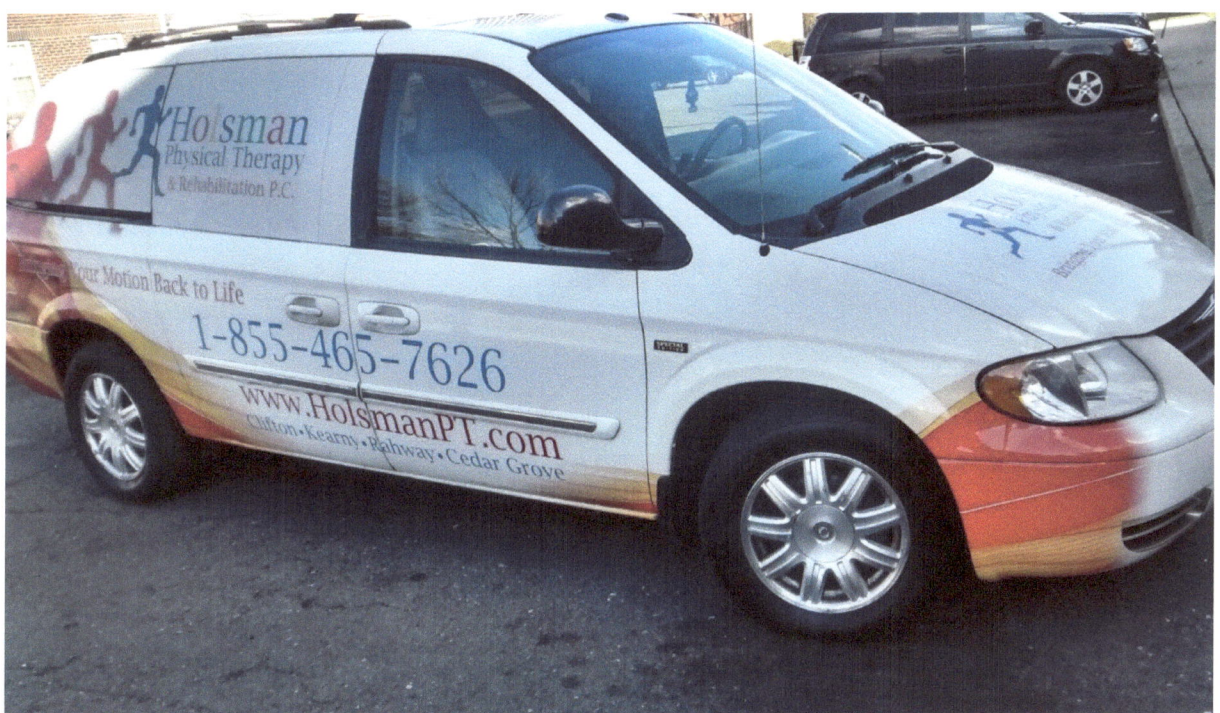

My first day for Physical Therapy was nice; I was really excited to start working out. They showed serious concern for everyone wanting to recover. They confirmed what time that they would be there, even ring the door bell and helped me into the van and taking me to therapy.

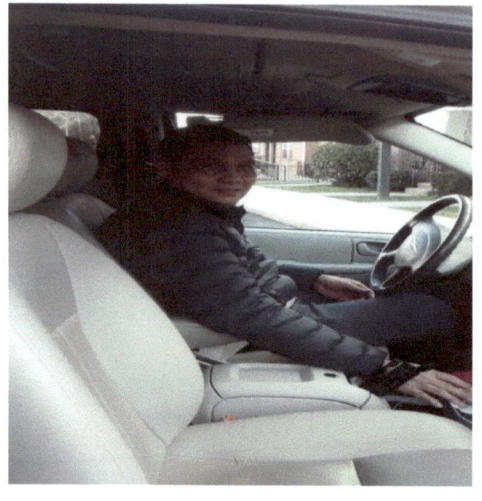 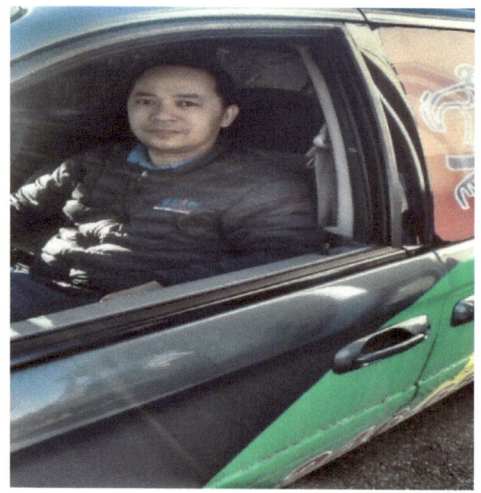

Mr.Nino   Mr.Francis

These are area's where I live and it is easy to get to Therapy in Kearny, where I'm very close to.

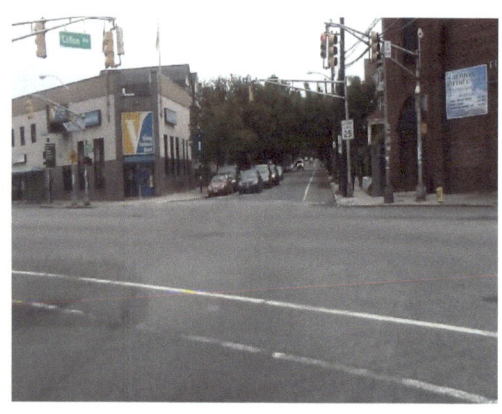 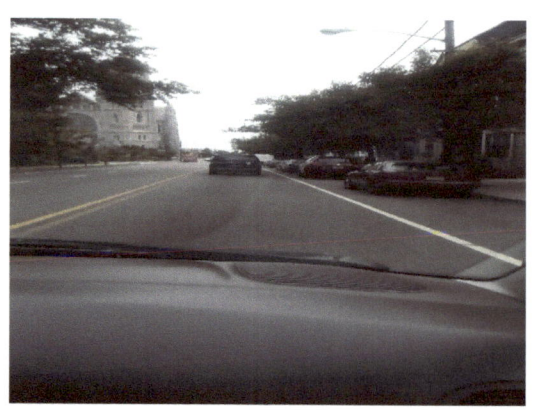

Very nice smooth riding back and forth from my destination.Sometimes one of the driver's put on some nice music of oldies and R&B. Many that they drive home sing to it, as they relax on the ride.

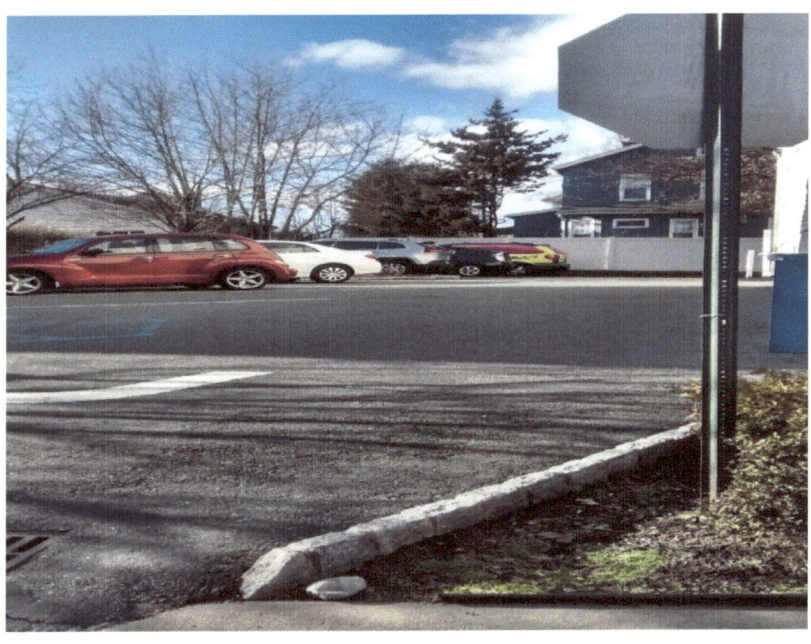

There is much parking for all to receive their first day of treatment as you can see.

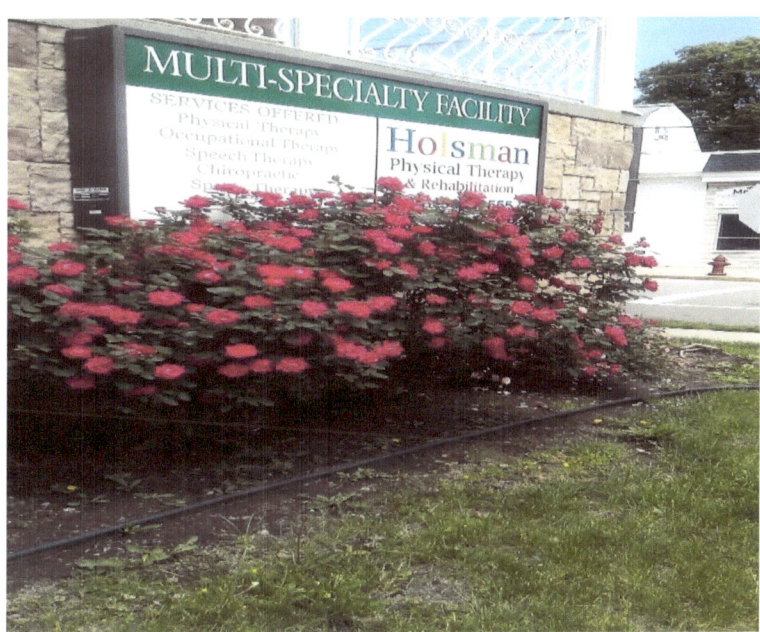

Well here we are, one of Holsman's Physical Therapy Recreational Centers.

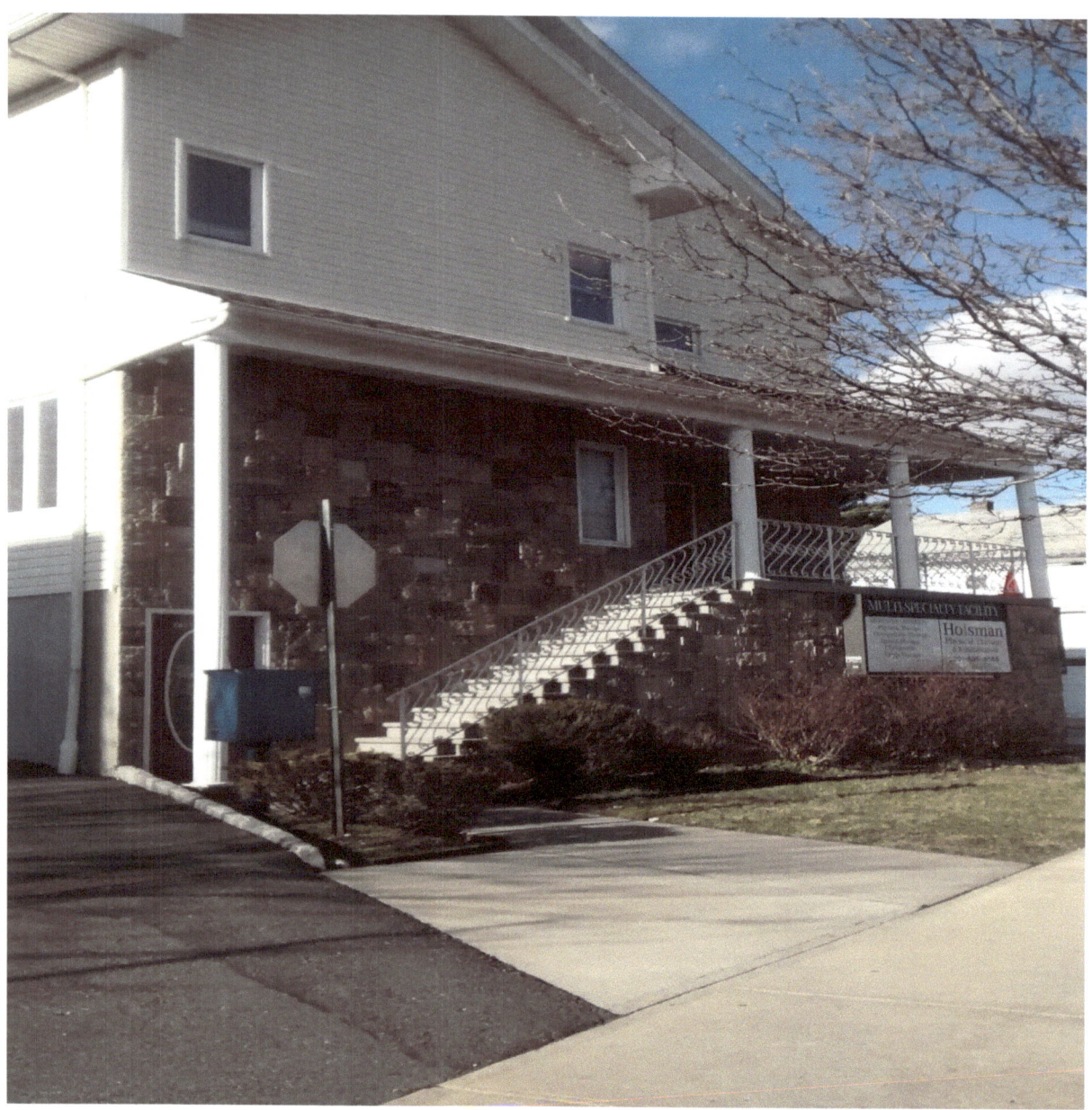

I knew this would be my second home, one beautiful place where I would learn how to walk again. That's what I felt as I entered with my wheel chair.

I knew this would be my second home, one beautiful place where I can recover ,

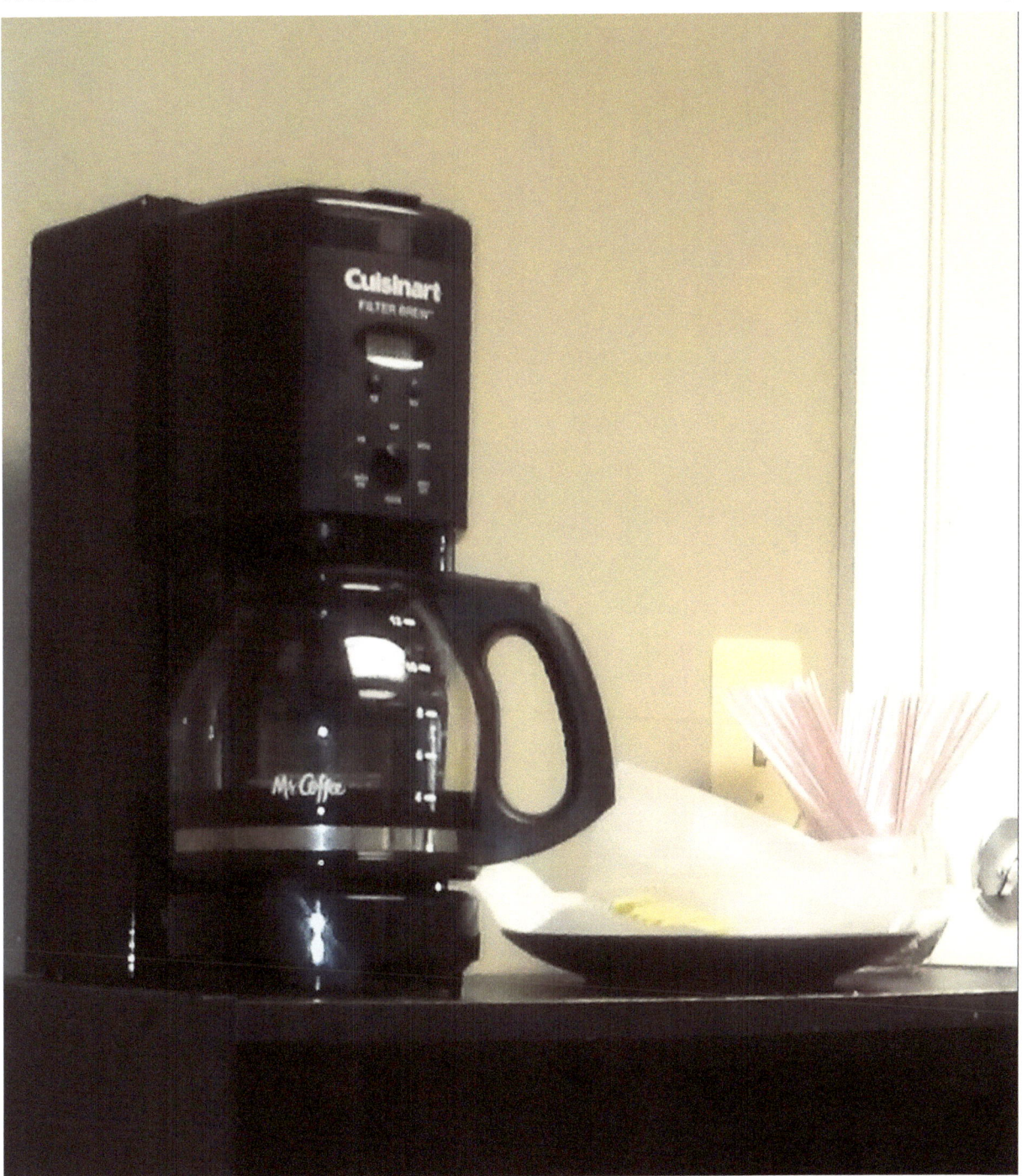

There a nice fresh cup of coffee everyday you come into Holsman's with even a healthy snack.

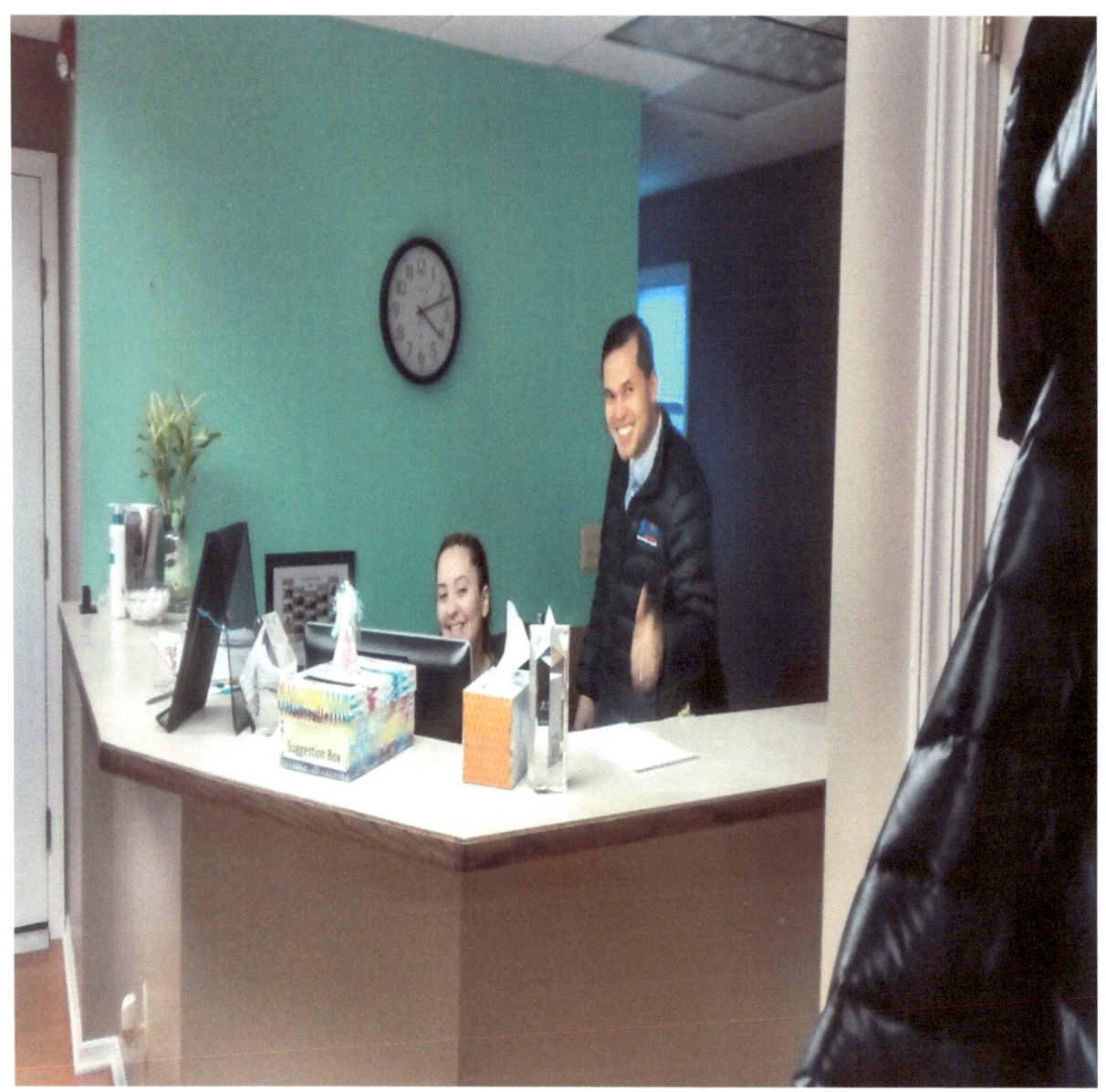

There's always a special greeting for all who enters therapy here at Holsman's. But this time it is from Mr. Richard Holsman CEO and Secretary Ms. Alicia sharing their welcome.

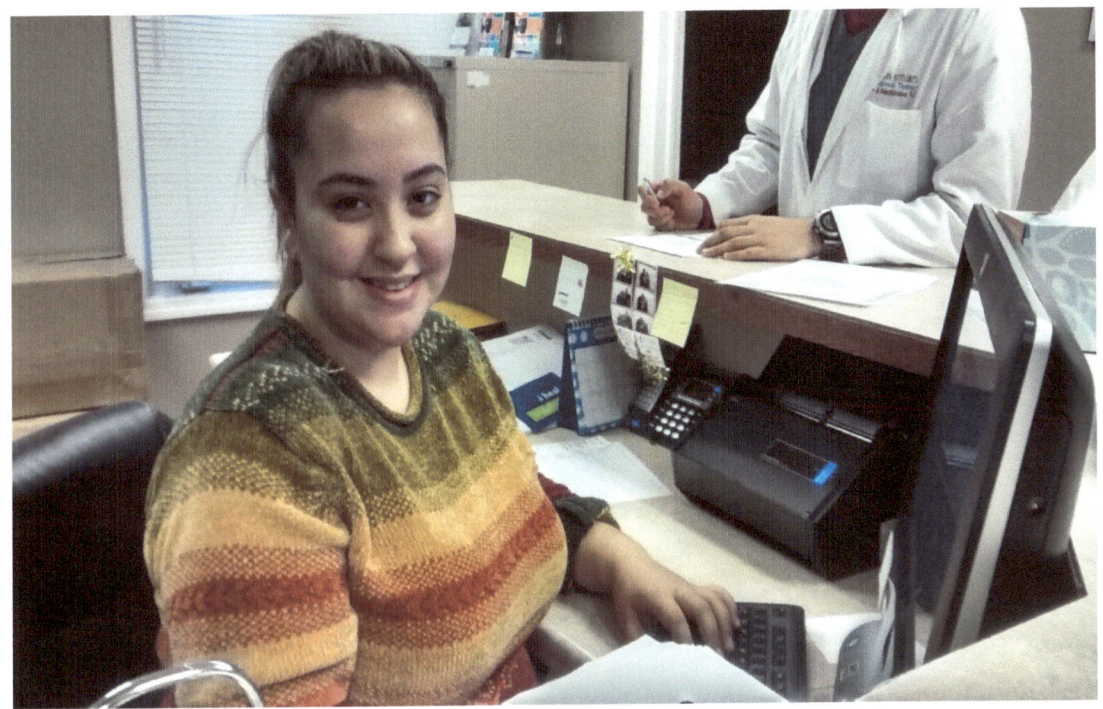

All the staff here is nice people in general, they had became something like a family that cares.

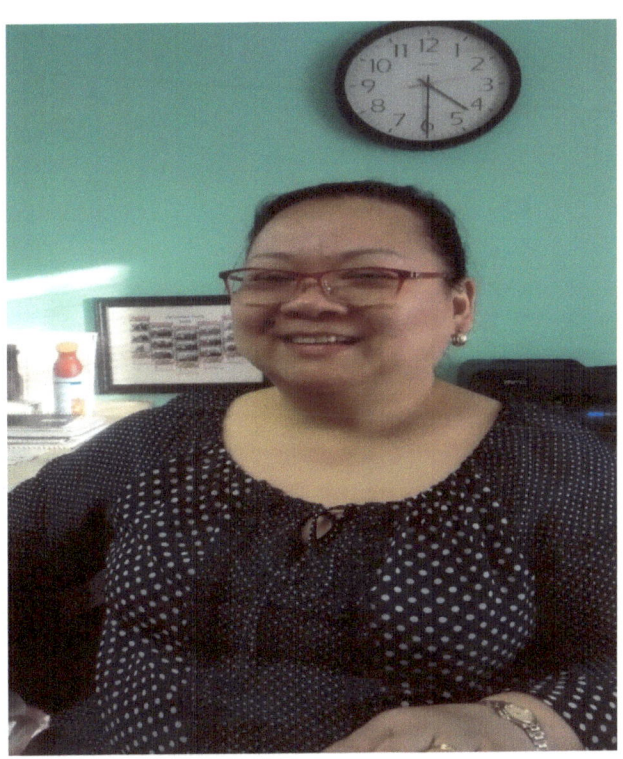

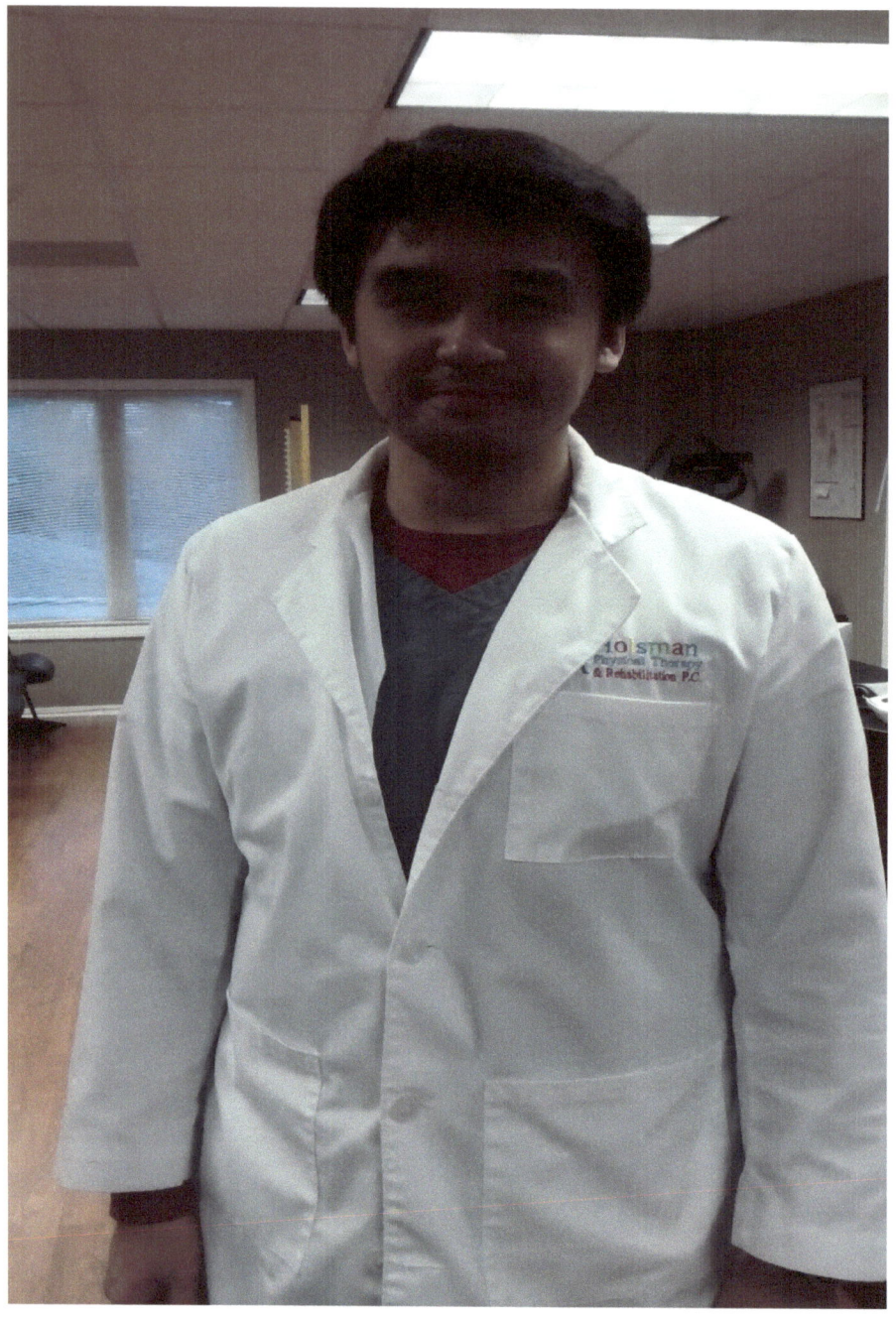

This is my main Coordinator Mr. Ben; I guess you can say that he is one of the main staff Holman's team that helped me start walking my first day for Physical Therapy was nice, I was really excited to start working out. They showed serious concern for everyone wanting to recover.

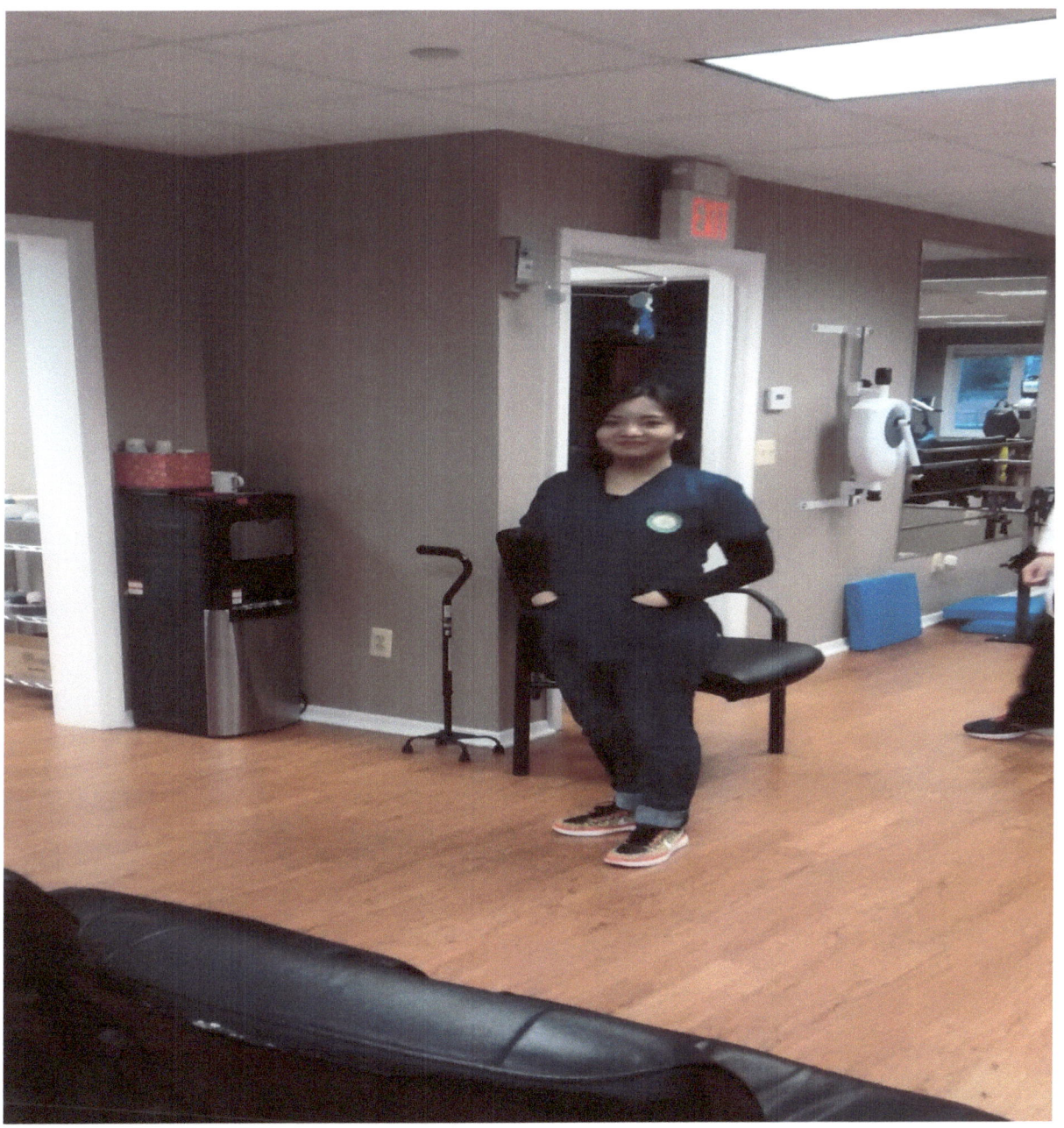

The staff here is very friendly and makes you feel comfortable. Asking questions like do you need anything, from heating pads, ice packs, water they really think about your health and care, and wish they can do more for you.

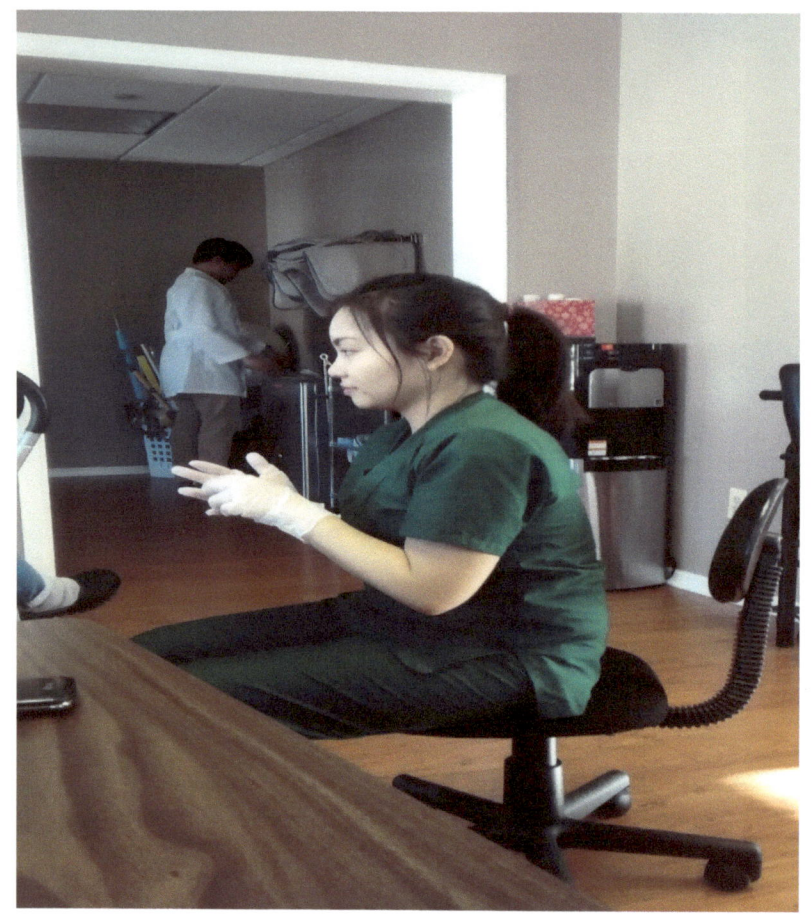

This is Ms. Fatima she also is staff therapist that always pushes me to do better and more.

This place is equipped with everything you'll need in your treatment plan, as you can see.

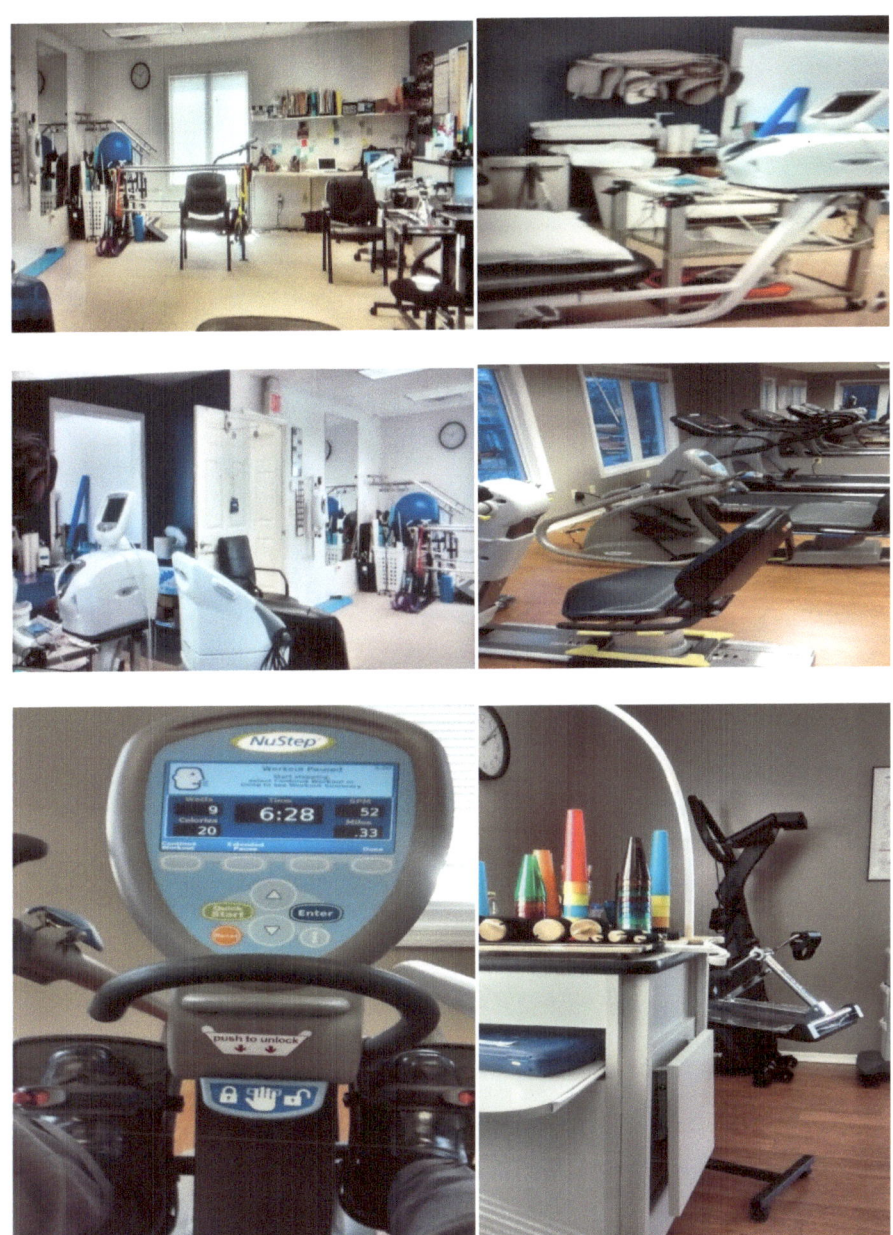

There is way more then you see here, just come and visit.

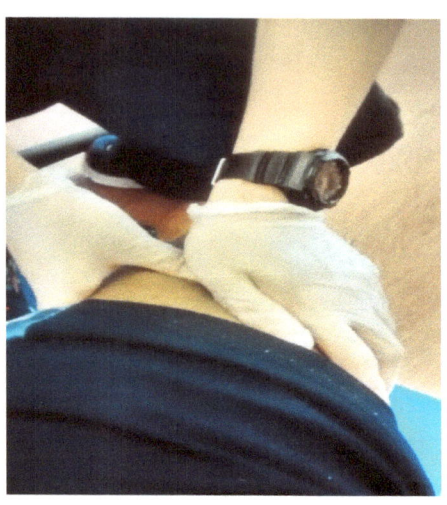

A little massage never hurt anyone

Sometimes this is I must, also a heat pad over you leg, even ice sometimes

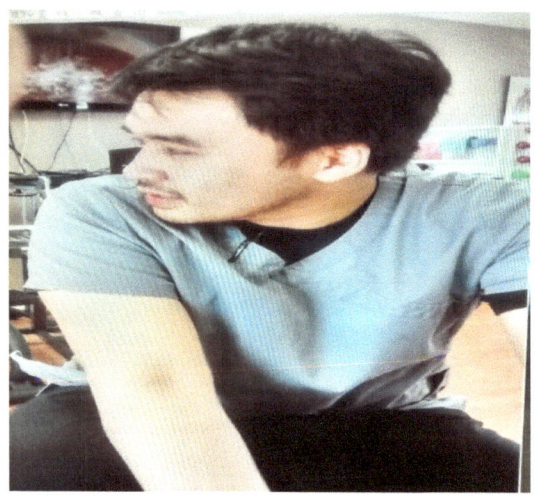

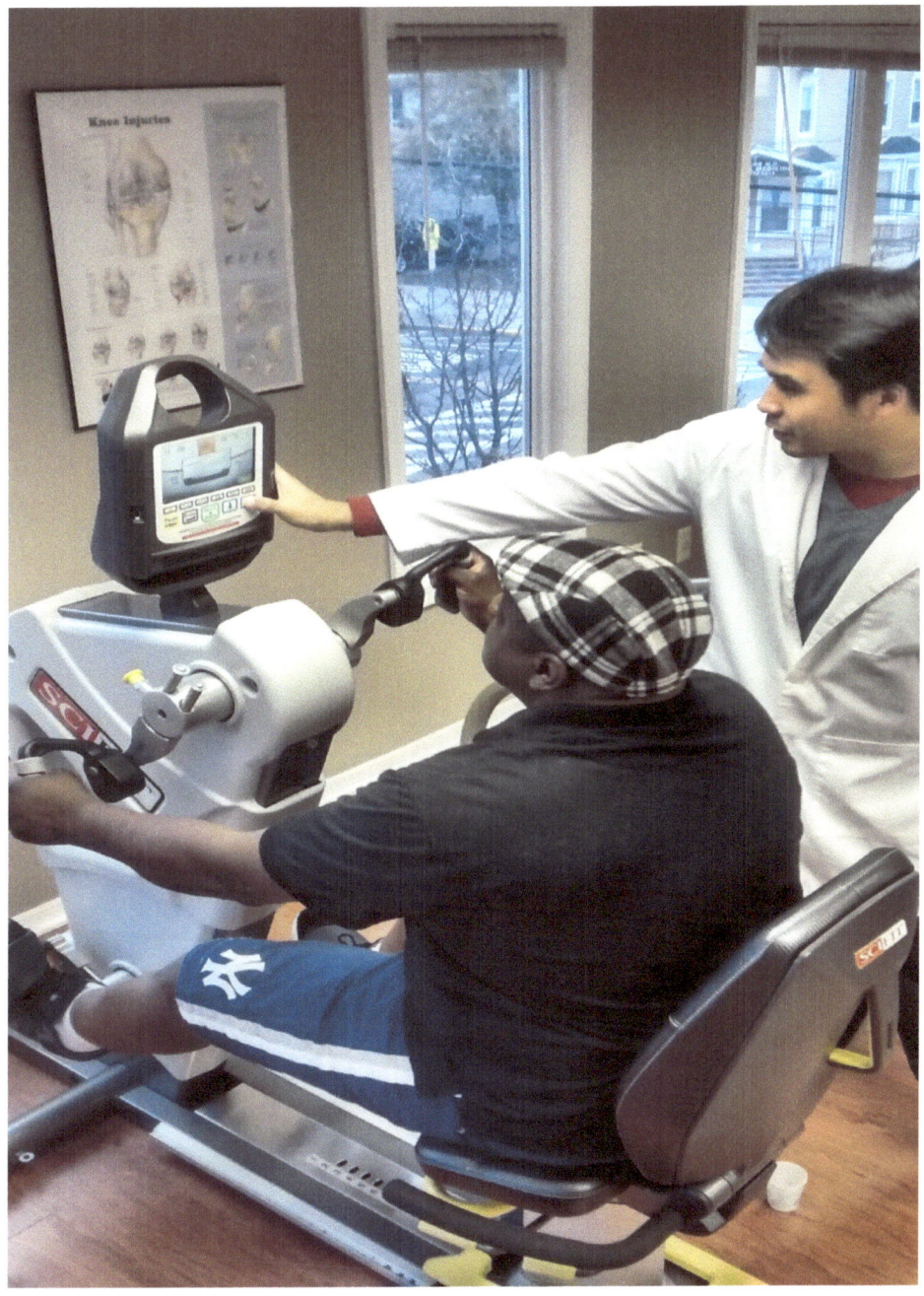

There are different levels on this bike, obstacles that are unreal.
I had to do fifth teen minutes on it, starting on level seven. By
not giving up my legs where getting stronger and better.

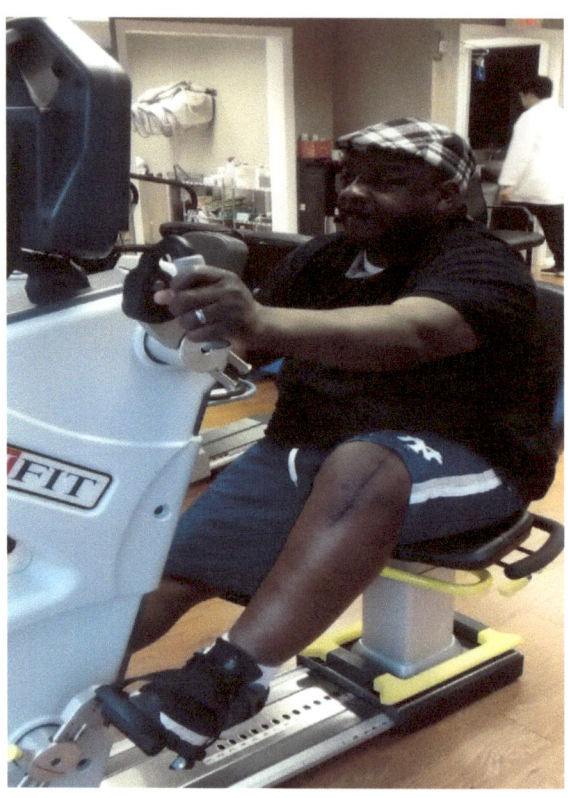

I started to really get into my therapy just as the coordinator suggested me to do.

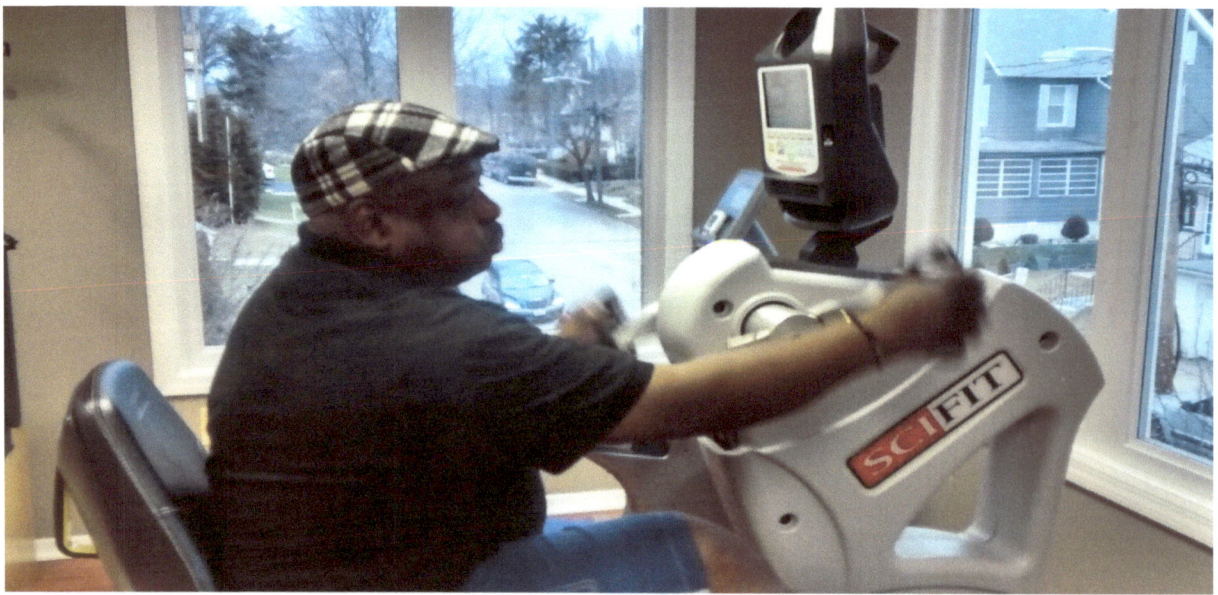

Tell you the truth it was hard and I made a dedication to myself to finish whatever I start.

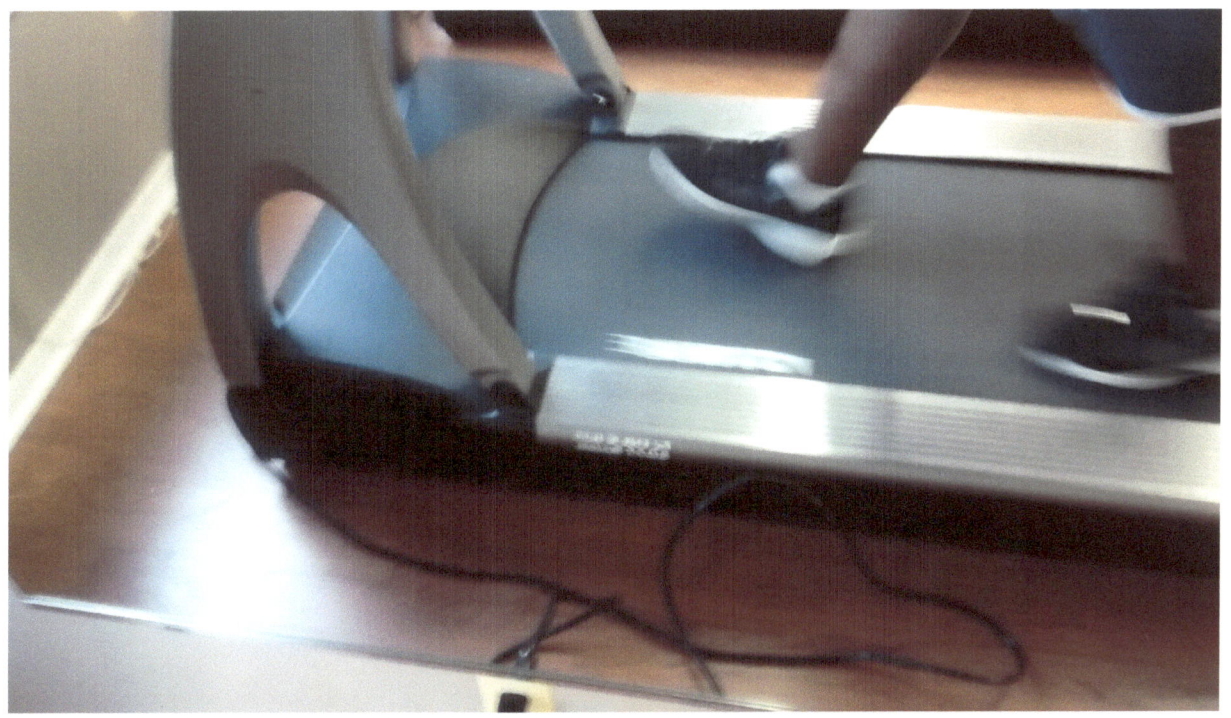

Feeling like the bionic man you can rebuild him.

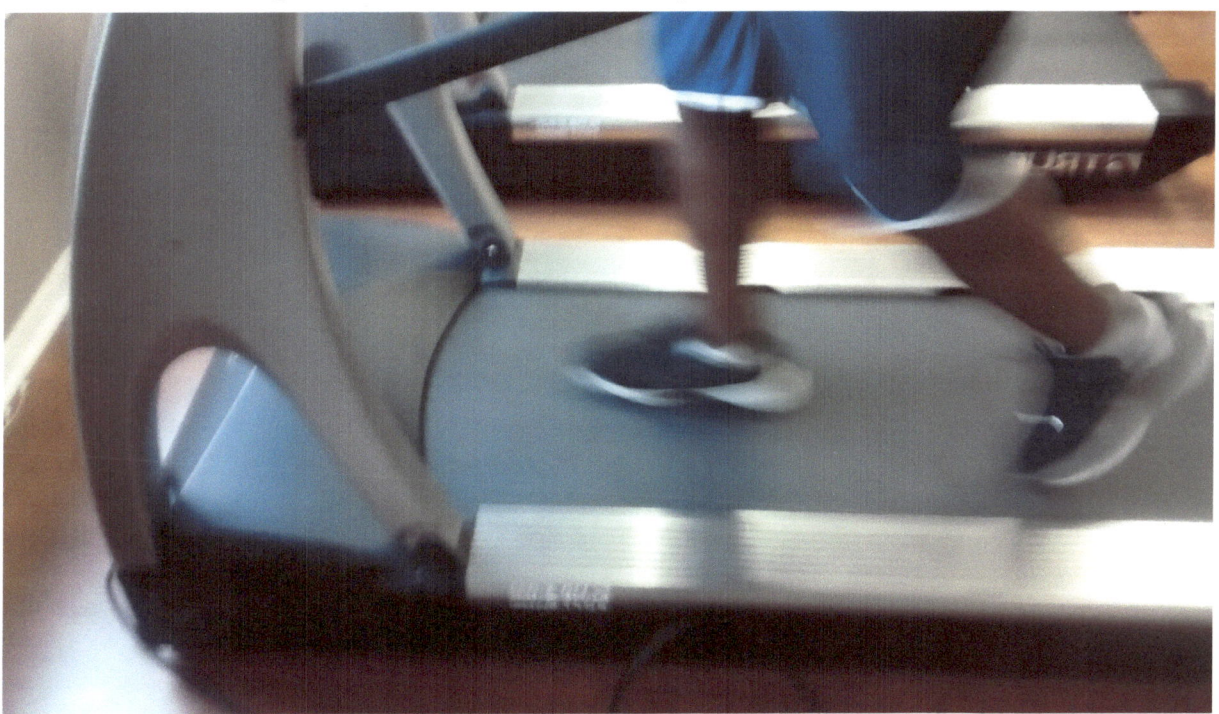

This was funny, but it helps my motivation.

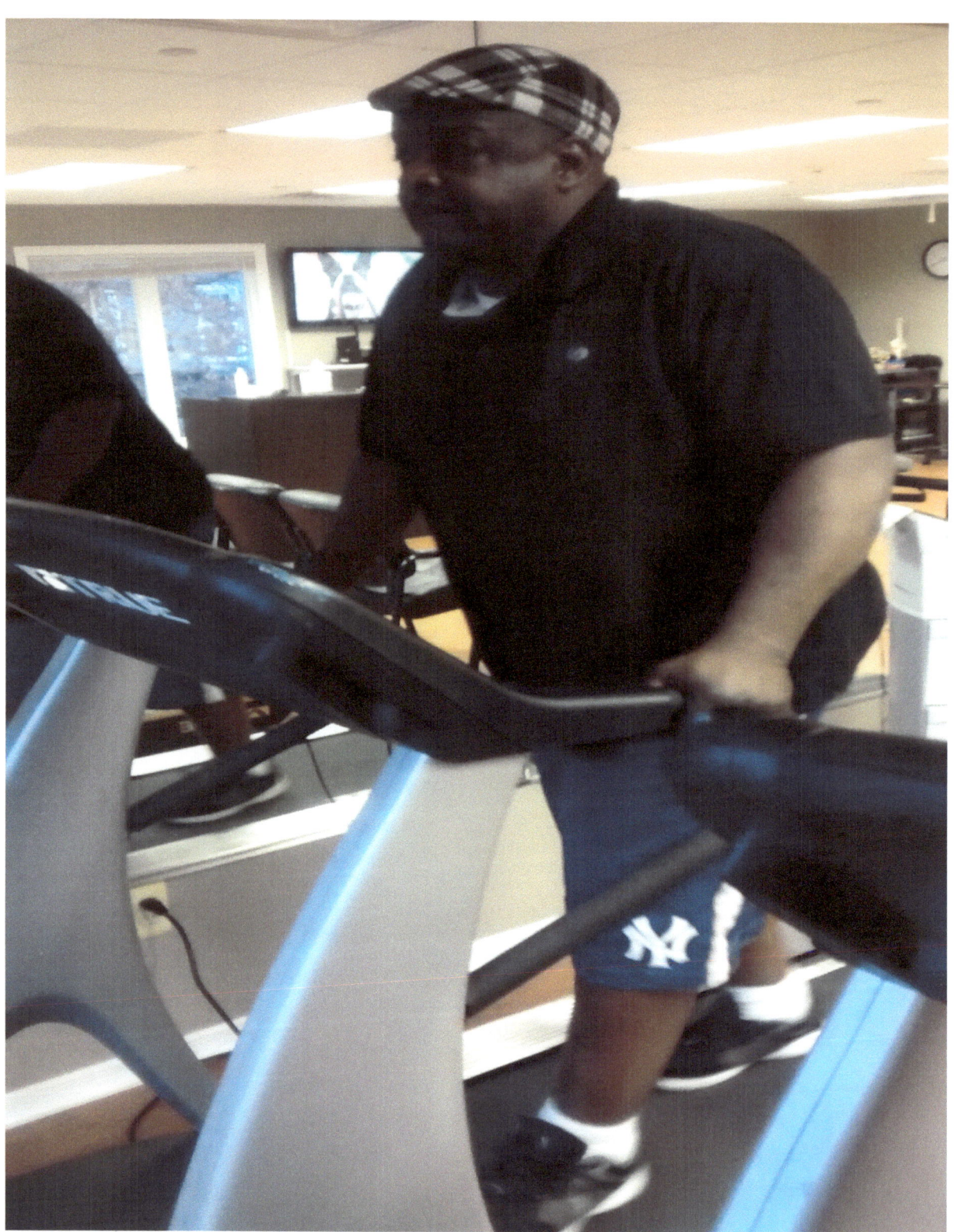

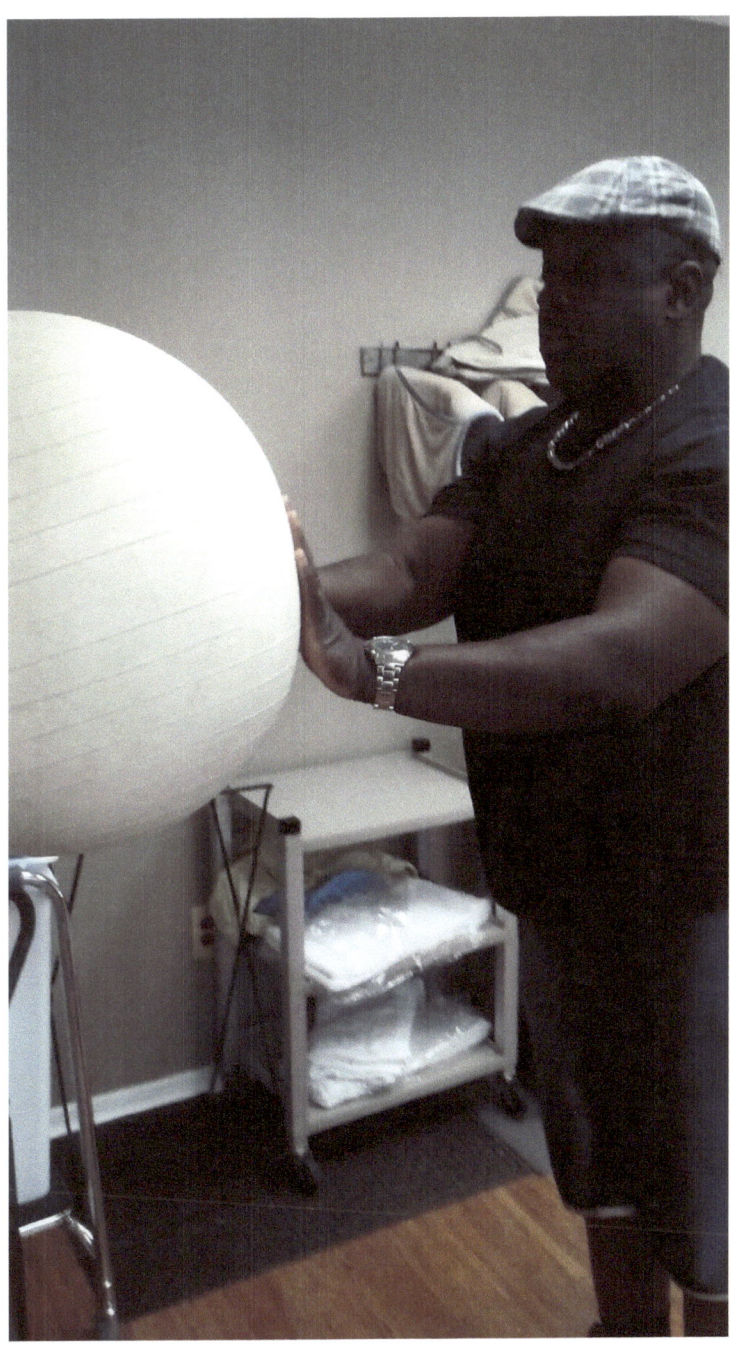

If you come for therapy and a workout trying to get better this is the place for you. I had lost weight and am continuing to reach more goals in my recovery to walk.

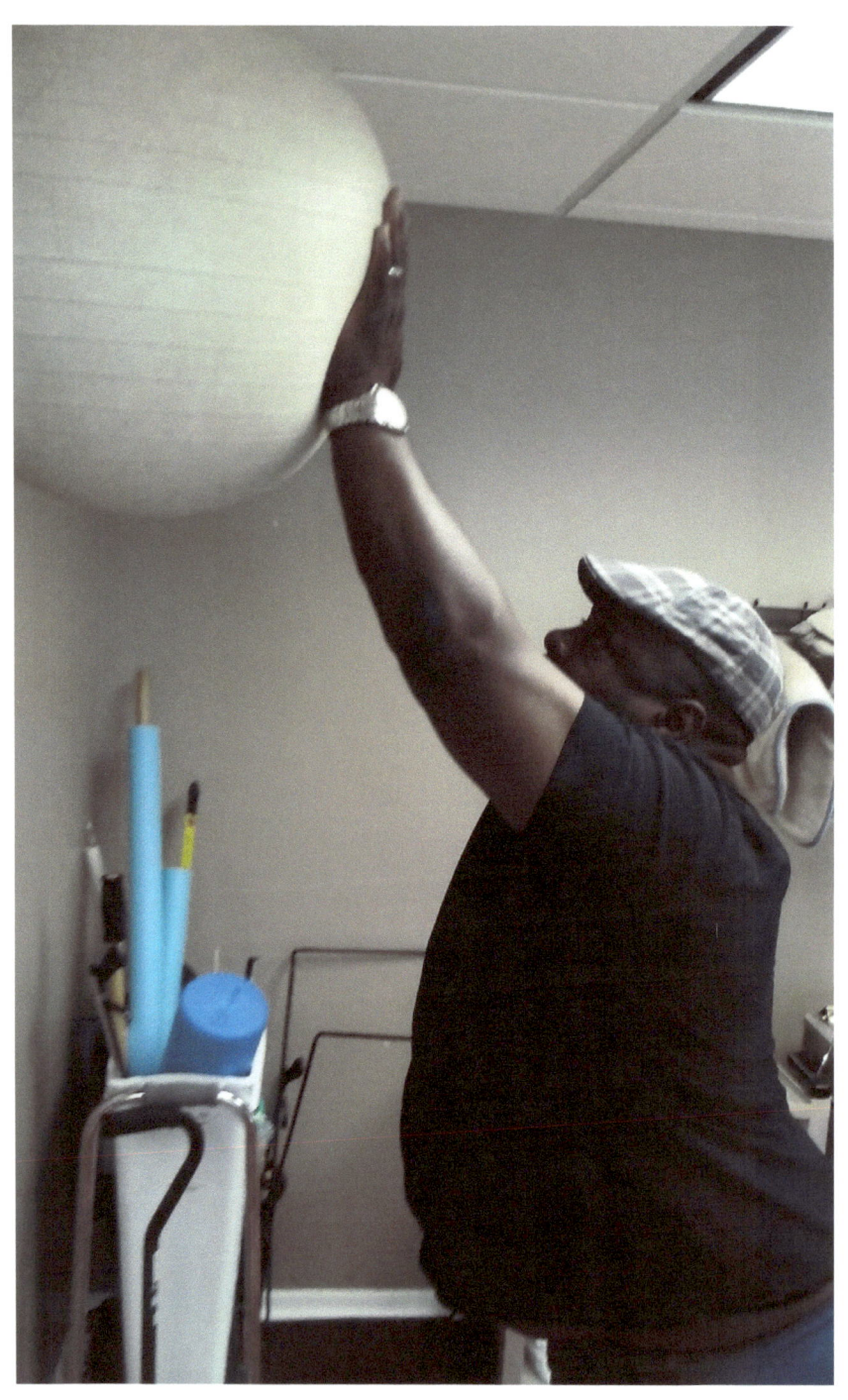

I even look different after each day of work out, the results will
show if you give it your all.

Something for you to expect, you feel much better than normal after a workout, relaxing at home, you really can sleep, like never before

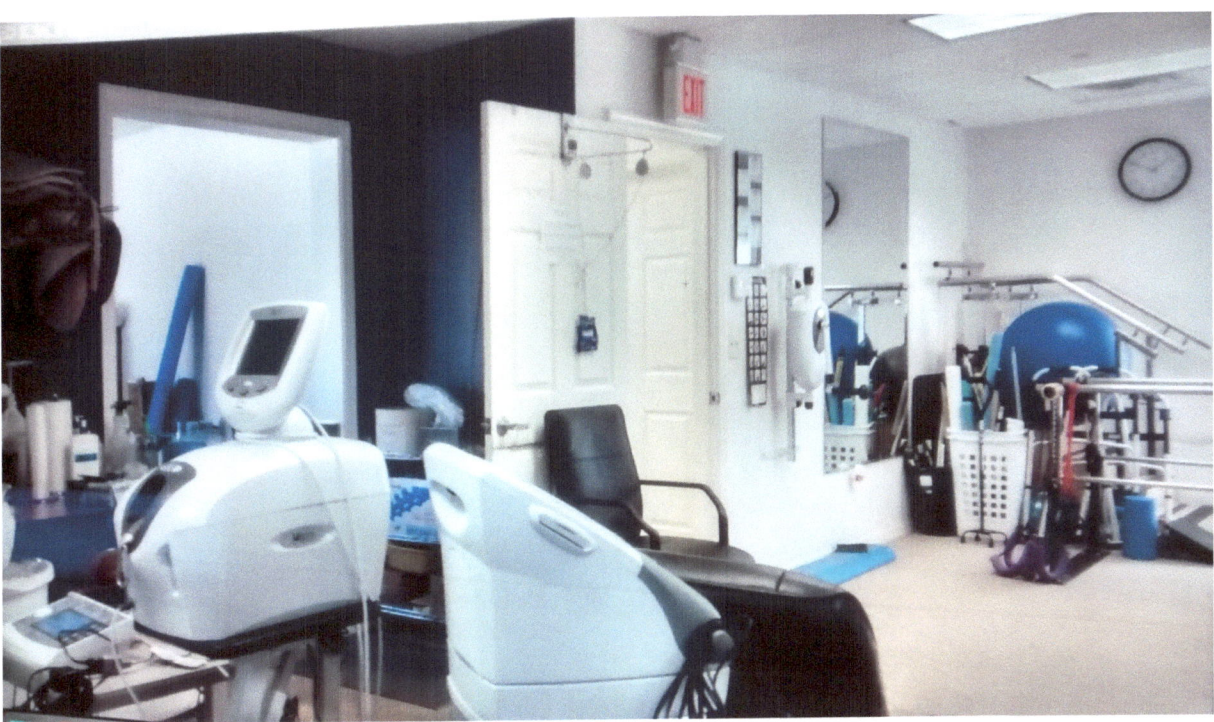

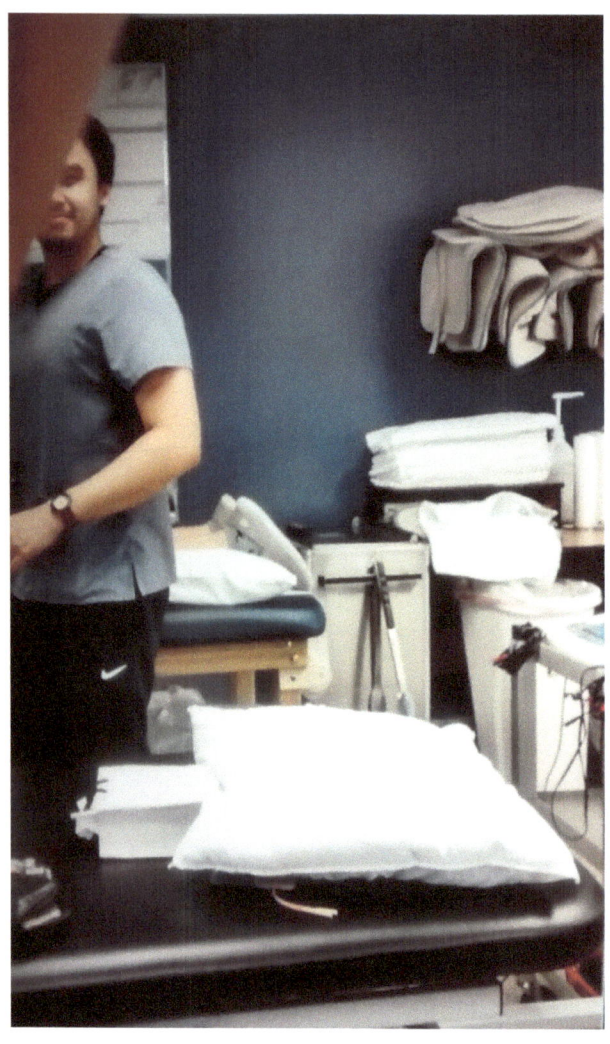

In this room you will get your leg to bend at a certain degree, but this is one of the most important parts of your therapy.

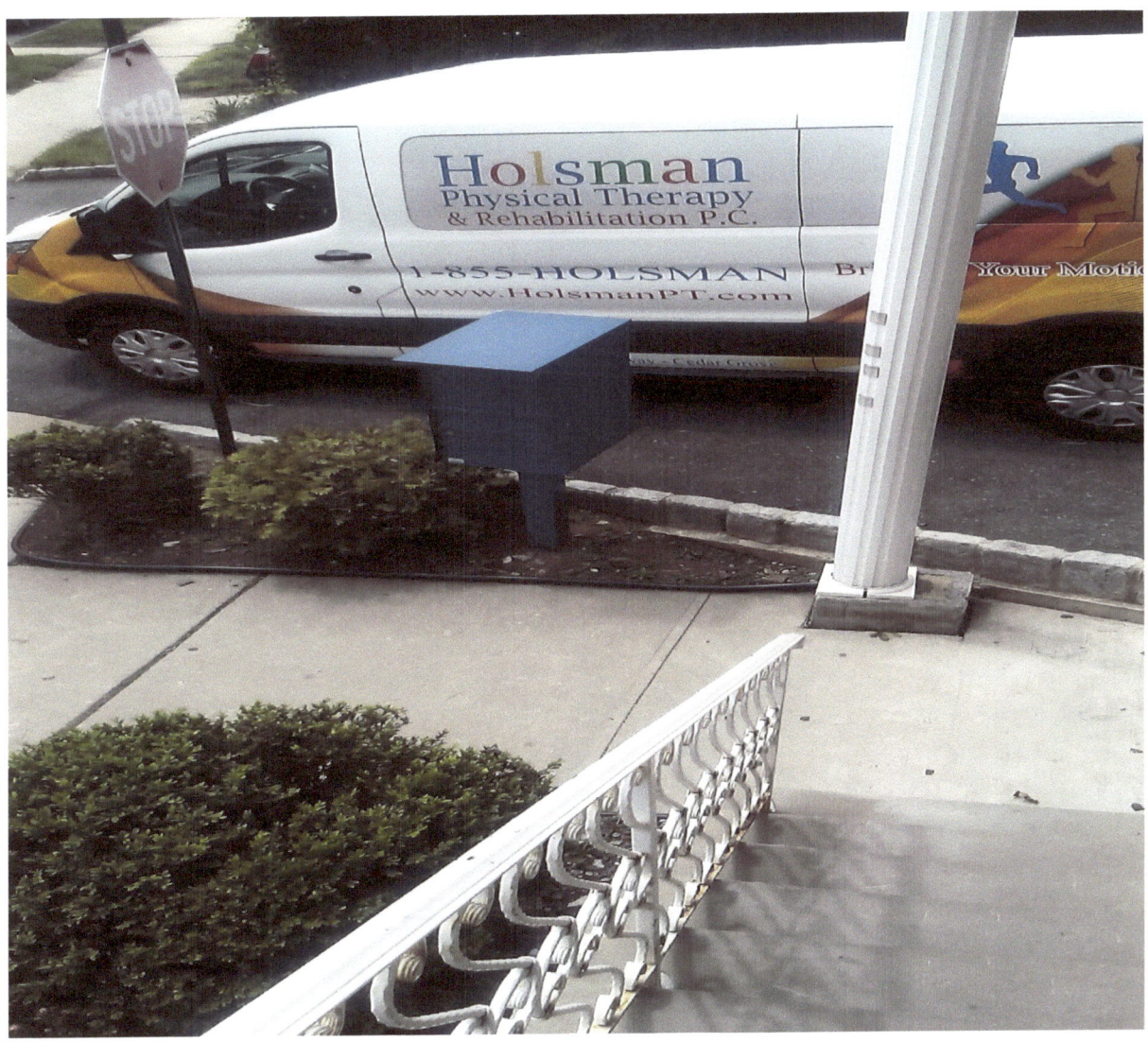

At this time I can walk up and down the stair easy, with no pain. I really respect Holsman's as my second family, through situations that I was going through and the determination to go on living my life as normal as possible.

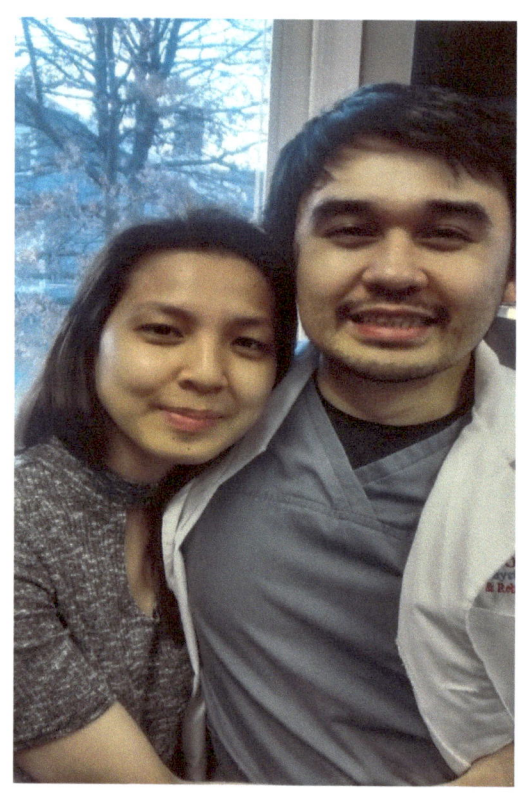

I know, I know, this is still family and also my therapy and this is how it worked for me.